# AETCOM

## Attitude, EThics and COMmunication

MANUAL

Learning Modules for MBBS Professional Year III
Competencies for the
Indian Medical Graduate

As Recommended by National Medical Commission

# AETCOM

## Attitude, EThics and COMmunication

MANUAL

Learning Modules for MBBS Professional Year III
Competencies for the
Indian Medical Graduate

As Recommended by National Medical Commission


**Nitin Ashok John**

MBBS MD FRSB (London, UK), FASSOPI (India), FAcad Med Edu (Cardiff, UK), FRSPH (London, UK 2021), PGDMLE (Medical Law and Ethics, NLSIU Bengaluru), DIH, PGDHA (Hospital Administration) MA (Public Administration), European Life Style Medicine Organization Certified Graduate

Professor and Head
Department of Physiology
All India Institute of Medical Sciences
Bibinagar, Hyderabad



CBSPD

**CBS Publishers & Distributors** Pvt Ltd

New Delhi • Bengaluru • Chennai • Kochi • Kolkata • Lucknow • Mumbai
Hyderabad • Jharkhand • Nagpur • Patna • Pune • Uttarakhand

**Disclaimer**

Science and technology are constantly changing fields. New research and experience broaden the scope of information and knowledge. The author had tried his best in giving information available to him while preparing the material for this book. Although all efforts has been made to ensure optimum accuracy of the material, yet it is quite possible some errors might have been left uncorrected. The publisher, the printer and the author will not be held responsible for any inadvertent errors or inaccuracies.

AETCOM
Attitude, EThics and COMmunication
MANUAL
Learning Modules for MBBS Professional Year III
Competencies for the
Indian Medical Graduate
As Recommended by National Medical Commission

ISBN: 978-93-5466-620-9



**First Edition: 2024**



Published by Satish Kumar Jain and produced by Varun Jain for
CBS Publishers and Distributors Pvt Ltd
4819/XI Prahlad Street, 24 Ansari Road, Daryaganj, New Delhi 110 002, India.
Ph: 011-23289259, 23266861 Website: www.cbspd.com
e-mail: delhi@cbspd.com

*Corporate Office:* 204 FIE, Industrial Area, Patparganj, Delhi 110 092, India
Ph: 011-4934 4934 Fax: 011-4934 4935 e-mail: publishing@cbspd.com; publicity@cbspd.com

***Branches***

- **Bengaluru:** Seema House 2975, 17th Cross, K.R. Road, Banasankari 2nd Stage, Bengaluru 560 070, Karnataka, India
  Ph: +91-80-26771678/79 Fax: +91-80-26771680 e-mail: bangalore@cbspd.com
- **Chennai:** 7, Subbaraya Street, Shenoy Nagar, Chennai 600 030, Tamil Nadu, India
  Ph: +91-44-26680620, 26681266 Fax: +91-44-42032115 e-mail: chennai@cbspd.com
- **Kochi:** 42/1325, 1326, Power House Road, Opposite KSEB, Power House, Ernakulam 682 018, Kochi, Kerala, India
  Ph: +91-484-4059061–67 Fax: +91-484-4059065 e-mail: kochi@cbspd.com
- **Kolkata:** 147 Hind Ceramics Compound, 1st Floor, Nilgunj Road, Belghoria, Kolkata 700 056, West Bengal, India
  Ph: +91-33-25633055/56 e-mail: kolkata@cbspd.com
- **Lucknow:** Basement, Khushnuma Complex, 7-Meerabai Marg (Behind Jawahar Bhawan), Lucknow 226 001, Uttar Pradesh, India
  Ph: +91-522-4000032 e-mail:tiwari.lucknow@cbspd.com
- **Mumbai:** PWD Shed, Gala No. 25/26, Ramchandra Bhatt Marg, Next to JJ Hospital, Gate No. 2, Opp Union Bank of India, Noorbaug, Mumbai 400009, Maharashtra, India
  Ph: +91-22-66661880, 66661889 e-mail: mumbai@cbspd.com

***Representatives***

- **Hyderabad** 0-9885175004
- **Jharkhand** 0-9811541605
- **Nagpur** 0-8692091830
- **Patna** 0-9334159340
- **Pune** 0-9664372571
- **Uttarakhand** 0-9716462459

*Printed at:* Mudrak, Noida, UP, India

# Preface

I am very happy to present *AETCOM* for Third MBBS Professional. The introduction of course on Attitude, Ethics and Communication as Learning Modules for MBBS students has strengthened the foundation of medical education for which National Medical Commission needs to be all appreciated. The medical students have to achieve professional expertise and to become competent doctors. It is not only the knowledge and competency which is required but a medical student's needs to be groomed to achieve clinical and communication skills as well. The book has been designed to inculcate high moral principle and ethical values.

The important topics which mark the uniqueness of the book is comprehensive coverage of topics such as foundations of bioethics, case studies on patient autonomy and decision making between doctor and patients in health care, medicolegal, sociocultural and ethical issues pertaining to refusal of care including do not resuscitate and withdrawal of life support. Medicolegal aspects in reference to consent and confidentiality and topic on empathy such as what does it mean to be family member of a sick patient. This book covers the curriculum and syllabus designed for students of MBBS as per recommendation of National Medical Commission. The book also covers important topics on medical ethics as recommended by Medical Counsils of various South Asian countries, UK, US, Canada, New Zealand and Australia. The key features of the book are that it has simplified text for easy reproducibility, it has well defined learning objectives at beginning of each chapter, it is written in easy, lucid and comprehensive language and it includes case scenarios for interactive learning and for better grasping of concepts. The manual is so designed that student can note lecture points; resolve case scenarios, write formative and summative assessment; and moreover after completion of the course a record is available to evaluate students performance and grade them.

I am thankful to Dr Vikas Bhatia, Director, All India Institute of Medical Sciences, Bibinagar, Hyderabad, for his encouragement and support. Mr Satish Jain (CMD) and Mr YN Arjuna (Senior Vice

President—Publishing, Editorial and Publicity), CBS Publishers & Distributors Pvt Ltd and all publishing staff.

I am thankful to my mother Mrs Ujwala Parekh, wife Dr Jyoti and son Joshua for all their support in this endeavor.

I hope that the book will stand immensely helpful to all the readers. All efforts have been made to write the script in flawless manner, and mistakes, if any, due to oversight may be pardoned. Looking forward for your suggestions to come up with the next edition based on your feedback.

**Nitin Ashok John**

# Contents

# Index of Competencies

Competency based Undergraduate Curriculum for the Indian Medical Graduate

***Competencies Addressed***

*The student should be able to:*

1. Identify, discuss and defend medicolegal, sociocultural, professional and ethical issues as it pertains to the physician–patient relationship (including fiduciary duty)
2. Identify and discuss physician's role and responsibility to society and the community that she/ he serves

*Reference:* AETCOM competencies for IMG; National Medical Commission; 2019

Module

3.1

# The Foundations of Communication

The most popular and in demand doctors are those who can communicate well. Acquiring a good communication skill is a prerequisite in delivering the best medical care to its patients. The present module is a step ahead of listening skills in communication which was taught in professional year II and "deals with impact of emotion in communication".

**Learning Objectives:** The student should be able to:

Demonstrate ability to communicate to patients in a patient, respectful, nonthreatening, nonjudgmental and empathetic manner.

## SESSION I: INTRODUCTORY SMALL GROUP SESSION (1 HOUR)

Key Points

### Recap of past learning

1. Communication is a key skill required to be mastered by medical students for gaining competency in delivering effective health care management.
2. The medical students need to be very patient while collecting information regarding patient's complaints, and moreover must address their patients with due respect in non-threatening and nonjudgmental manner. The genuine concern for addressing patients suffering and need should be the primary goal.
3. The essential qualities that will help medical students in developing clinical communication skills are patient listening, genuine concern for patient's agony and health issues, and their eagerness, interest and readiness to acquire the needed skills.
4. Effective communication will help the learners to understand and know their patient better, develop a good rapport with patients, understand patient's

perspective especially pertaining to their misconceptions, fears and worries and eventually build the patients confidence and trust on the doctor.

5. The Kalamazoo consensus statement describes the various essential elements of communication in medical encounters being faced by the medical professionals. A conference to discuss the above issue was organized by the Bayer Institute for Health Care Communication and the Fetzer Institute in the year 1999.

   As per the recommendation of the committee; the physician–patient communication is important in delivering effective health care services. The committee recommended formulation and implementation of effective communication-oriented curricula in medical education. The seven essential sets of communication were identified by the task group and these included:

   a. Build sound doctor–patient relationship;
   b. Plan methodology for communication for recording medical history;
   c. Gathering appropriate information while recording patient history of illness;
   d. Communication to know patient's perspective;
   e. Communication for information sharing with patients;
   f. Communication for arriving at common consensus regarding the patients health issue and management; and
   g. Providing closure to the discussion.

6. **Communication, Purpose and Modes of Communication**

## PURPOSE FOR COMMUNICATION

The main purpose for communication in hospital setting is for:

1. Recording the clinical history of patients.
2. Informing patients regarding his health status and available treatment modalities.
3. To health educate and counsel the patient and building their trust.
4. For developing rapport with the patient and building their trust.
5. Receiving patient's feedback.
6. Solving patients queries.

   **The various modes of communication include:**

   (a) Verbal communication, (b) Nonverbal communication, (c) Written communication, (d) Visual communication

7. **Developing Basic Skills for Effective Patient Centric Communication:** The key responsibilities of the teaching clinicians are to ensure that the students learn the art of effective communication.

8. The modalities of effective patient centric communication ensure that:
   a. Approach is patient centered.
   b. Patient should be given time for expression.
   c. The patients should not be an active listener only.
   d. Understanding patients ideas, worries and concerns. This will also help understanding the patient's expectation from treating doctor.
   e. Empathy towards patients.
   f. Developing personal rapport with patient.
9. The key components of effective communication strategies include:
   a. Self Introduction of oneself to the patients so that they are aware of expertise of doctors.
   b. Developing rapport with patients.
   c. Developing optimistic, caring, respectful and positive interpersonal behaviors.
   d. Active listening to patients.
   e. Empathy with patients in all situations.
10. Communication and challenging occasions to be addressed in hospital setup include:
    a. Delivering sad news to patients relative especially that of death of patients.
    b. Information regarding critical condition of patient to the patients.
    c. Communication with upset patient or patient's relative in OPD/IPD.
    d. Discussing regarding treatment modalities and cost of treatment especially to the poor patients.
    e. Communicating with hearing impaired patient.
    f. Communicating with patient or their relatives after receiving negative feedback regarding the treatment which was given.

## EMOTIONS AND COMMUNICATION

1. The medical doctor is looked as a savior by his patients for relief from their illness and sufferings. In such a context a doctor needs to maintain their emotional compose, be calm and

maintain poise, be cheerful, have patience listening to patient's complaints, be empathetic towards the patients and provide the best available care as expected of his/her competency level. Hence, it is very necessary that doctors have suitable emotional intelligence which is earmarked by one's ability to monitor his own and others' feelings and emotions so as to effectively discriminate the emotional input and thereof take appropriate thinking and action.

2. The trainee doctors should be groomed to improve their emotional vocabulary, as well made aware of using appropriate verbs and adjectives while expressing their thoughts to the patients because the words, facial expressions and body language expressions have a deep impact in understanding their physical health conditions as well provide solace to them for an early recovery from the ailments.
3. As doctors are also at receiving end after sharing their thoughts; they should be able to appraise expressions of emotions of their patients in themselves and their responses should be communicatively expressed. This art of comprehending others emotion and getting the expression of same feeling in oneself may help learn becoming empathetic.
4. The empathetic nature in doctors is vital in patients recovery as this has great social and physical implications such as it boost physiological effects on human body like lowering stress levels, makes person emotionally happy, lessens anxiety and helps developing optimism and psychological and mental wellbeing.
5. Any patients who report for hospitalization usual carry negative emotion as they have fear and are worried regarding their health and recovery.
6. In such situation such as hospitalization it was observed in various research settings that a neutral but optimistic toward responses towards patients query (regarding his health profile and management) and apprehension builds confidence in patient to disclose their health issues in totality and this helps the doctor to give best medical care with tailored treatment plans.
7. Empathy and sympathy shown by doctors are factors which influence patient for accepting the recommended line of treatment. This helps in building rapport and due trust in the doctor.

8. Empathy may get affected and eroded over period of time as doctor may find difficulty in balancing distancing and connecting with patients due to bust schedule. But doctors should devoting time in building trust of patient apart from delivering standard medical care.
9. Catering to emotional needs of patients is good for patient's recovery, good for doctors for understanding patients mental status to cope up with disease and as this will facilitate prognosis of patient as well as it will good for repute of the hospital.

## BIBLIOGRAPHY


1. Adams K, Cimino JE, Arnold RM, Anderson WG. Why should I talk about emotion? Communication patterns associated with physician discussion of patient expressions of negative emotion in hospital admission encounters. Patient Educ Couns 2012 Oct;89(1):44–50.
2. Bowman D, Cushing A. Ethics, law and communication. In: Kumar P, Clark M, (Eds.) Kumar and Clarke's Clinical Medicine. 9th ed. Philadelphia, PA: Elsevier;2017:Chap 1.
3. Bukstein DA. Patient adherence and effective communication. Ann Allergy Asthma Immunol 2016;117(6): 613–9.
4. Crozier WR. Blushing and the Social Emotions: The Self Unmasked (New York: Palgrave Macmillan, 2006).
5. Emotional Intelligence and Its Impact on Communication in the Workplacehttps://franchetti.com/emotionalintelligence-impact-communication- workplace/ October 11, 2016.
6. Empathy in medicine. https://www.cma.ca/physician-wellness-hub/content/empathy-in-medicine
7. Evans, D. Emotion: The Science of Sentiment (New York: Oxford University Press 2001:5–6.
8. Gilligan T, Coyle N, Frankel RM, et al. Patient clinician communication: American Society of Clinical Oncology consensus guideline. J Clin Oncol 2017;35(31):3618–32.
9. Hausberg M. Enhancing medical students' communication skills: development and evaluation of an undergraduate training program. BMC Medical Education 2012;12:16.
10. Kotchemidova C. "Emotion Culture and Cognitive Constructions of Reality," Communication Quarterly 58, no. 2 (2010): 207–34.
11. Nitin Ashok John, Jyoti Elgiva John Effective Communication Skills Facilitates Better Health Care Delivery Br J Pharm Med Res 2022 Jan-Feb.;7(1):3527–32.

12. Rime B. "Interpersonal Emotion Regulation," in Handbook of Emotion Regulation, James J Gross (Ed.), New York: Guilford Press 2007:466–68.
13. Salovey P, Alison Woolery, John D Mayer. "Emotional Intelligence: Conceptualization and Measurement," in Blackwell Handbook of Social Psychology: Interpersonal Processes, Garth J. 1 O. Fletcher, Margaret S Clark (Eds.), Malden MA: Blackwell 20011:279–307.

## SESSION II: FOCUSED SMALL GROUP SESSIONS (2 hours)

**Goal:** Focused small group session with role play where the students have an opportunity to observe, criticize and discuss common mistakes in doctors way of dealing with emotions.

**Activity**

1. The students are divided among groups with 10 student members in each group.
2. The students are told to enact a role play in reference to goal mentioned as above with doctor addressing a patient.
3. An alternate group of 10 students will observe the role play and students shall observe, criticize and discuss common mistakes while dealing with emotions.

   **Note:** Both group will enact a role play alternatively and so also comment on ideal situations and criticism of role play.

**Role Play 1 (Participant Group 1: Ex Roll Nos 1–10)**

**Mimicked Venue** Jubilee Hills Nursing Home

**Doctor** Mr Ram Lingam—please come in

**Mr Ram Lingam** Doctor I am having pain in abdomen and become intense after eating food, well many a times I have delayed lunch at 4 pm

**Doctor** If you have any addictions

**Mr Ram Lingam** I want to tell you that when I was in Xth standard, I started chewing beetle nuts, well I was not a very good students, I used to watch movies with friends, I liked freaking on weekends... My neighbor Mr Raju was a drunkard.

**Doctor** Please stop such long stories Mr Ram Lingam, just tell if you smoke or take alcohol ... Don't you see my busy OPD ... Well

**Mr Ram Lingam** Yes Sir but just wanted to tell that in my college days I use to booze, another incidence of ...

**Doctor** Oh ... Oh...

**Doctor** Scribbles some medicine … and ask patient to go.

**Mr Ram Lingam** Doctor my ... oh I am afraid of my pain … don't know … when it will go ... well doctor what about precaution … my diet ...

**Doctor** Calls for next patient … Well Mr Ram Lingam you seem to be a cator … good dramatist … ask query to nurse pleas ... please go

**Write your opinion about the role play regarding doctor's consideration towards patient. How you as a doctor respond in such situation.**

**Observation by (Participant Group 11: Ex Roll Nos 11–20)**

An alternate group of 10 students to observe the role play and observe, criticize and discuss common mistakes in doctor's way of dealing with emotions. The students shall discuss and record their opinion below:

The group teacher/facilitator to make opinion regarding student's presentation. The students to note important clues and corrective action below: **Ideal situational modification in such scenario:**

**Role Play 2 (Participant Group 11: Ex Roll Nos 11–20)**

**Dr Naidu** Hello Mr Reddy; I Hope all well in family, seeing you after long time, well I am your family doctor, I know you and all in family for last 20 years.

**Mr Reddy** I am having pain while passing urine and I have burning sensation too.

**Dr Naidu** Well Mr Naidu … You always seem to be worried ... just drink ample water.

**Mr Reddy** Doctor twice in last week there was blood in my urine …

**Dr Naidu** I hope you are not seeing any horror movies Mr Reddy these days.

**Mr Reddy** Sir I cannot sleep and have a frequent urge for passing urine. **Dr Naidu** is busy texting some information to his friend and he ... neglects Mr Reddy's conversation.

**Mr Reddy** I vomited twice yesterday and ...

**Dr Naidu** See Reddy you just drink ample water, don't watch horror movies and may be see you later.

**Mr Reddy** Please prescribe some medicines, please I am anxious and worried.

**Dr Naidu** Doctor his busy chatting in mobile ... Well Mr Reddy Bye ... Stop being emotional

**Mr Reddy** Doctor but ... If ... again ... if

**Dr Naidu** Scribbles some medicine, handover chit to patient and gets up and walk out his OPD ...

**Observation by (Participant Group 1: Ex Roll Nos 1–10)**

An alternate group of 10 students to observe the role play and observe, criticize and discuss common mistakes in doctor's way of dealing with emotions. The students shall discuss and record their opinion below:

## EXERCISE 1

Students are instructed to go through the paper and describe the importance of emotion in communication for effective health care delivery and record their findings here.

Link–Paper—Adams K, Cimino JE, Arnold RM, Anderson WG. Why should I talk about emotion? Communication patterns associated with physician discussion of patient expressions of negative emotion in hospital admission encounters. Patient Educ Couns. 2012 Oct;89(1):44–50.

## SESSION III

Skills lab sessions where students can perform tasks on standardized or regular patients with opportunity for self critique, critique by patient and by the facilitator.

## EXERCISE 1

**Explaining prognosis to patient**

**Doctor** The patient is of HIV and has pulmonary Koch

**Nurse** Sir I have ask the patient to get tested for viral load

**Doctor to Nurse** Let me inform patient

**Patient** I am feeling hopeless so severe diseases ... my patients sobs ... I am really sad and depressed ... what will happen to me ... which medicines to be taken.

**Doctor** My goodness ... you patient just want we doctors to dance to your emotion ... You are unwell ... You either will recover or will die ... what worst can happen ...

**Relatives** Doctor, do not be so rude ...

**Doctor** Well see I cannot spend all time in convincing you and pacifying you ...

**Doctor to Nurse** We are seeing patient dying ... these patients want to keep them pacifying ... who has so much of time ...

**Point of inaction during above role play:**

1. One participant each will be doctor, nurse, patient, nursing attendant and two patients relatives (two students to direct the role play and two students to play role of self critique)
2. One facilitator to overall coordinate, guide and opine.

   The students to write the complete enacted role story, opinion as self critique, patient's critique comments and facilitator comments below.

## EXERCISE 2

**Communicating and recording a case history of patient of hypertension with considering importance of emotion in communicatin.**

**Action:** Small group task for students: They should enact a small play where doctor needs to be empathetic and understanding to the patient and also responds to their emotions and apathy with optimist communication.

1. Two students to record patients illness history as doctor.
2. Two observer students can be self critique who shall assess the pitfall in effective communication.
3. Two observer students to interact with patients in effective, empathetic, nonjudgmental and nonthreatening way to record patients history.
4. Facilitator to opine and conclude the sessions.

The students to write the enacted interaction, opinion of self critique, patient's critique comments and facilitator comments below:

Disclaimer: All information in chapter (**Module 3.1: The Foundations of Communication 3**) includes but not limited to; and is for information purpose only. The author declares that the sincere attempt has been made to give standard accurate information in the chapter, but it is not a substitute for any legal or professional advice. The reader should seek advice from legal professional if they are seeking consultation and advice for any issue associated with fiduciary duty.

**Students Assessment by Faculty In charge**

1. **Formative:** Participation in session 2 and performance in session 3 may be used as part of formative assessment.

**Name of Student:**

Participation in session 2:
Excellent/Very Good/Good/Satisfactory/Poor

**Signature:** Faculty In-charge AETCOM

Participation in session 3:
Excellent/Very Good/Good/Satisfactory/Poor

**Signature:** Faculty In-charge AETCOM

2. **Summative:** May be deferred.

Module

3.2

# Case Studies in Bioethics: Disclosure of Medical Errors

**Background:** This module introduces the student to full disclosure of mistakes. The case study discussed in the chapter is self designed for giving insight regarding the topic. The teacher can formulate case study from practical experience or live situation in their setup for teaching concepts to the student.

**Learning Objectives:** The student should be able to: Demonstrate an understanding of the implications and the appropriate procedure and response to be followed in the event of medical errors.

## ANCHORING LECTURE (1 hour)

Implications of medical error and responses for resolving them:

### Key Points

1. Medical errors in medical practice as doctors may occur as doctors being human may unintentionally make medical error in judgment while treating cases.
2. The doctors may at times do not make full disclosure of medical error to patient. This is not a good practice and doctors should accept the responsibility of error, learn from the mistake and do needful compensation if any, as per law and provision prevailing.
3. Assessment of risk factors which may lead to medical errors is necessary for prevention of any future occurrence and so also for delivering quality health care.
4. Medical errors may have a negative impact on doctors, nurses as well as hospital administrative staff and they may have feeling of guilt, distress, fear and disappointment.

5. In a hospital; the modeling of error acknowledgement and regular discussions regarding measures for error ratification is must and especially; this benefits resident doctor and junior consultants in addressing medical errors.
6. The complete information regarding cause of medical error and provisions in cases of damage must be informed to patients and their families. But the disclosure to patients or their relatives is usually limited.
   a. Doctors in consultation of the head must identify cause of medical error before informing relatives.
   b. Following which the patient's relatives are to be called.
   c. Calmed down and gradually explained the occurred medical error.
   d. Doctor responsible for same should accept the accountability.
   e. Pacify relatives and inform them regarding reason for the occurrence of medical error, how the same will affect the patient's health and information regarding the measures to be taken to repair injury.
   f. Patients relatives must be assured that all possible will be done to correct the medical error.
   g. Law of compensation should be informed to patient's relatives.
   h. Arrange for completing protocol for compensation existing as per provision in Code of Ethics.
7. Opening communication about medical errors to patients and their families is a challenging situation for doctors as they fear for wrath of family members of patient and also of law and provisions of penalty under Consumer Protection Act.
8. Death audit which is being conducted in hospitals do help in identifying medical errors and help to generate vital information for prevention of such mistake in future.
9. The occurrence of medical errors can only be reduced if there is establishment of standard transparent medical errors reporting protocol designed for doctors/health care providers, storing the same information in centralized repository, reviewing the error reports and planning strategies for future medical care so as to provide detailed feedback to health care providers.
10. The disclosure of medical errors is acknowledged in codes of professional medical ethics. Moreover any attempt to provide full disclosure is compromising autonomy and right of informed consent of patients.
11. Limited disclosure at times leads to patient distrust and matter is challenged in court for suing the doctors.
12. Apology for medical error in proper framework of words may at times resolve the probable lawsuits. But mostly doctors feel that apology means excepting fault and this may lead to litigation and at times doctor have to pay financial compensation too.
13. To lower malpractice claims for medical error and negligence and for sustenance of faith in doctor its better than medical care provider avoid 'shame and blame' game and accept accountability for action.

## BIBLIOGRAPHY

1. A view of Medical Negligence and Medical Error in India. https://www.legalserviceindia.com/legal/article-690-a-view-on-medical-negligence-and-medical-errors-in-india.html
2. Bari A, Khan RA, Rathore AW. Medical errors; causes, consequences, emotional response and resulting behavioral change. Pak J Med Sci 2016 May-Jun;32(3):523–8.
3. David P Lind, David R Andresen, Andrew Williams. Medical Errors in Iowa: Prevalence and Patients' Perspectives. J Patient Saf 2020 Sep;16(3):e199–e204.
4. Hobgood C, Peck CR, Gilbert B, Chappell K, Zou B. Medical errors—what and when:what do patients want to know? Acad Emerg Med 2002;9(11):1156–61.
5. Hobgood C, Xie J, Weiner B, Hooker J. Error identification, disclosure, and reporting:practice patterns of three emergency medicine provider types. Acad Emerg Med 2004;11(2):196–9.
6. Jennifer J. Robertson, Brit Long. Suffering in Silence: Medical Error and its Impact on Health Care Providers. The Journal of Emergency Medicine 2018;54(4):402–9.
7. Kalra J, Massey KL, Mulla A. Disclosure of medical error: policies and practice. J R Soc Med 2005 Jul;98(7):307–9.
8. Kronman AC, Paasche-Orlow M, Orlander JD. Factors associated with disclosure of medical errors by housestaff. BMJ Qual Saf 2012; 21(4):271–8.

**Disclaimer:** All information in chapter **(Module 3.2: Case Studies in Bioethics: Disclosure of Medical Errors)** includes but not limited to; and is for information purpose only. The author declares that the sincere attempt has been made to give standard accurate information in the chapter, but it is not a substitute for any legal or professional advice. The reader should seek advice from legal professional if they are seek consultation and advice for any issue associated with disclosure of medical errors.

## ASSIGNMENT I: INTRODUCTION OF CASE (1 hour)

The teacher must introduce the case to the students. The task may be carried in small groups and instruct the students to study the case.

**Case:** After examining Nikhil for a abrasion injury due to brushing of hand against a pointed nails of door gate, doctor advices nurse to load TT injection. Doctor continues seeing cases due to heavy rush of patient in his OPD and after 10 minutes he remembers that he has to give injection TT to Nikhil. He goes to injection room but nurse is not in room, he takes the loaded syringe and administers the injection and asks the patient to wait for his abrasion injury. Doctor returns and continues seeing patient. After Nurses come and inform doctor that she has loaded TT for Nikhil. Doctor is in shock and ask the nurse which injection was loaded earlier, the nurse informs that it was metoclopramide injection for Nilesh. By the time Nilesh developed extrapyramidal symptoms and signs of torticolis. The doctor further gets patient admitted for observation.

**Points for discussion:**

1. Medical errors in clinical care.
2. The correct approach to disclosure of medical errors.
3. Consequence of failure to disclosure of medical errors including medicolegal, social and loss of trust.

## ASSIGNMENT II: SELF-DIRECTED LEARNING (2 hours)

The students should browse and study the following research papers for self-directed learning and write the observations below.

1. Hobgood C, Peck CR, Gilbert B, Chappell K, Zou B. Medical errors—what and when:what do patients want to know? Acad Emerg Med 2002;9(11):1156–61.
2. Hobgood C, Xie J, Weiner B, Hooker J. Error identification, disclosure, and reporting:practice patterns of three emergency medicine provider types. Acad Emerg Med 2004;11(2):196–9.
3. Kronman AC, Paasche-Orlow M, Orlander JD. Factors associated with disclosure of medical errors by housestaff. BMJ Qual Saf. 2012;21(4):271–8.
4. Bari A, Khan RA, Rathore AW. Medical errors; causes, consequences, emotional response and resulting behavioral change. Pak J Med Sci. 2016 May-Jun; 32(3):523–8.
5. David P Lind, David R Andresen, Andrew Williams. Medical Errors in Iowa: Prevalence and Patients' Perspectives. J Patient Saf. 2020 Sep;16(3):e199–e204.

## OBSERVATIONS

## ASSIGNMENT III: ANCHORING LECTURE (1 hour)

The students should write the notes below. Points for lectures are discussed at beginning of chapter

## ASSIGNMENT IV: DISCUSSION AND CLOSURE OF CASE (1 hour)

**Points for discussion:**

1. Medical errors in clinical care.

   Doctor should have been careful while instructing for loading injection to nurse, he should have himself gone to injection room, checked the TT vial, check expiry, get it loaded and administer the same.
2. The correct approach to disclosure of medical errors.

   Doctor should explain the error of giving metaclopramide injection instead of TT. Doctor should keep patient in observation well at this stance there is lesser chances of any complications.

   The correct approach to disclosure of medical errors may be followed as below:

   a. Doctors must identify the act of medical error before informing relatives.
   b. Following which the patient's relatives are to be called.
   c. Calming down patients relative they should be explained the occurred medical error.
   d. Doctor responsible for same should accept the accountability.
   e. Pacify relatives and inform them regarding reason for the occurrence of medical error, how the same will affect the patient's health and information regarding the measures to be taken to repair injury/or complications if any.
   f. Patients relatives must be assured that all possible will be done to correct the medical error.
   g. Law of compensation should be informed to patients relatives.
   h. Arrange for completing protocol for compensation existing as per provision in Code of Ethics.
3. Consequence of failure to disclosure of medical errors including medicolegal, social and loss of trust.

   **Medicolegal Consequence:** Penalty on Doctor depends on whether it was a civil negligence or criminal negligence. Whether the act of commission was that of a gross neglect, slight neglect or ordinary neglect decide the nature of offence. Civil may include financial compensation to be paid while criminal negligence includes imprisonment or penalty such as temporary/permanent withdrawal of practicing license, etc. [**Note:** Criminal negligence includes loss or harm cause to individual to extent of injury and death.]

### Social Impact on Doctor

Doctor may develop sense of guilt, depression, fear and stress and this may lead to burnout of doctors working capacity, post-traumatic stress disorders or chances of suicidality.

**Trust:** There will be loss of patients trust.

> **Disclaimer:** All information in chapter (**Module 3.2: Case Studies in Bioethics: Disclosure of Medical Errors)** includes but not limited to; and is for information purpose only. The author declares that the sincere attempt has been made to give standard accurate information in the chapter, but it is not a substitute for any legal or professional advice. The reader should seek advice from legal professional if they are seeking consultation and advice for any issue associated with fiduciary duty.

### Assessment

1. **Formative:** The students may be assessed based on their active participation in the sessions including role play on disclosure of errors.
2. **Summative:** Write short notes on

**1. What is the ethical standard in dealing with medical errors?**

Module

3.3

# The Foundations of Communication

**Background:** Communication is an important skill to be acquired by a doctor for successful professional carrier. This module is a continuation of learning art of effective communication skills as emphasized earlier. The module emphasis on administering informed consent especially in context to surgical procedure. The case study discussed in the chapter is self designed for giving insight regarding the topic. The teacher can formulate case study from practical experience or live situation in their setup for teaching concepts to the student.

**Learning Objectives:** The student should be able to:

1. Communicate to patients in a respectful, nonthreatening, non-judgmental and empathetic manner.
2. Explain medicolegal, sociocultural and ethical issues pertaining to consent for surgical procedures.
3. Obtain informed consent and appropriately address patient queries undergoing a surgical procedure in a simulated environment.

Introductory small group session on the principles of communication with focus on administering informed consent especially pertaining to consent for surgical procedures.

**Key Points**

1. Surgical consent is a progressive event of communication that starts from preoperative stage and progresses to perioperative, and postoperative stage.

2. Obtaining informed consent for any surgical procedure is an ethical and legal prerequisite.
3. Informed consent is promoting the right of autonomy, shared decision making protocol and providence of patient-centered care.
4. Certain elements of surgical consent need better answer especially pertaining to issues if a patient's preoperative consent covers the post-operative complications occurring if any? if a patient relative who is a surrogate decision maker refuse such treatment which patient has consented for or vice versa accept when it was refused by the patient and extent to which the surrogate decision making being accepted in case of surgeries.
5. Surgeons opine that when a patient consent for surgery it is expected that he/she has implicitly consented for the treatment and expected complications. But rightfully consent for treatment, risks, foreseen complications and management of all these complications must be obtained in a go.
6. The obtainment of inadequate informed consent is usually considered a tort of medical negligence.
7. Informed consent entrusts patient with right to autonomy and right of self-determination regarding their own health.
8. A written consent usually obtained for a patient is a legal prerequirement but every surgeon should communicate and as well as document communication regarding proposed surgery, reasons for the procedure, expected complications, available management alternatives and probable risk and complication of them too.
9. Nowadays, patient's consent (or patient relatives who are surrogate decision maker) is required prior to any diagnostic and therapeutic interventions, except in emergency condition such as threatening infectious condition which endangers community health.
10. Implicit and intrinsic to the principle of consent for treatment is the refusal option for patient or their surrogate.
11. During surgical intervention the treatment modalities may change as per outcome of surgery and hence informed consent may be reobtained if there are changes in plan of management. Thus, the process of getting informed consent is patient-centered decision making process.
12. The components of legal consent are that patient should be mentally sound and in position to make decision regarding the decision of health care, they should be able to understand treatment modalities available and benefit and risk of these, that patient can understand the information provided to them regarding their health care and can arrive at a rational decision making and finally patient is able to communicate the same to doctor.

13. Its doctors duty that patient be provided detailed adequate information regarding his health, patient must consent regarding acceptance of treatment freely with his own free will without any threat or coercion and even consent regarding the patients treatment should be obtained by the doctor.
14. All dialogues regarding consent process should be recorded and documented safely.
15. If a patient or surrogate refuses a treatment, the doctor should explain to the patient or surrogate as case may be the various complications which may arise due to refusal of surgery and even warn them that death can occur in such consent is obtained for anesthesia and surgery regarding all foreseen situations.
16. It is important to remember that as any complications can occur in course of surgery and surgeon might require performing an additional surgical procedure; hence consent for the same is necessary to be obtained from patient prior to surgery. Similarly consent should be obtained for mechanical ventilation support in case of unexpected unforeseen situation. The patients must also authorize some person of his family to act as surrogate decision maker in case on unforeseen circumstances and the patient has been landed up in incapacitated position. The surrogate must be aware of choices, values and preferences of patients.
17. Naming a surrogate by patient for making decision on patient's treatment and management in case of patient becoming in capacitated may be carried out meticulously. Moreover the surrogate who is authorized on legal basis is being entrusted authority to make medical decision as enjoyed by the patient under sanctity of legal rights. .
18. If patients due to his in capacitated condition lose the capacity to make decision and has not ear marked any surrogate decision maker then patients relative are expected to act as surrogate decision maker by the doctor.
19. Thus, to conclude the practices in obtaining consent for surgery must be a continuum process from preoperative, perioperative and postoperative period. It should involve constant discussion with patient/surrogate in a joint decision-making manner. The patient's values and health goals and health expectation must be known by surgeon so as it will help in providing better medical care. Identifying a surrogate decision maker prior to surgery can be termed as good clinical practice. A decision and consent regarding unforeseen circumstances should be done in advance. Moreover, surgeons communication should always be of hopeful and optimist to build trust of patient and surgeon should respect patient/surrogate decision if they feel to obtain palliative treatment instead of aggressive interventions but the surgeon should decide the course of management in best interest of patient's health.

## BIBLIOGRAPHY

1. Berg JWAppelbaum PJ Informed Consent: Legal Theory and Clinical Practice. 2nd ed. New York, NY Oxford University Press Inc 2001.
2. Brock DW The ideal of shared decision making between physicians and patients. Kennedy Inst Ethics J 1991;128–47.
3. Choudhry NK, Choudhry S, Singer PA. CPR for patients labeled DNR: the role of the limited aggressive therapy order. Ann Intern Med 2003;13865–8.
4. Cohen S. The nocebo effect of informed consent. Bioethics. 2014;28: 147–54.
5. Gert HJ Avoiding surprises: a model for informing patients. Hastings Cent Rep 2002;32(5):23–32.
6. James L. Bernat, Lynn M. Peterson. Patient-Centered Informed Consent in Surgical Practice. Arch Surg 2006;141(1):86–92.
7. Kurt E, Ucar M, Atac A. Quality of an informed consent prior to a surgical intervention? Experience of a teaching hospital Pak. J Med Sci 2016;32:206–10.
8. Lidz CW. Informed consent: a critical part of modern medical research. Am J Med Sci 2011;342:273–5.
9. Mazur DJ. Why the goals of informed consent are not realized: treatise for informed consent for the primary physician. J Gen Intern Med 1988;3370–80.
10. McClung JA Time and language in bioethics: when patient and proxy appear to disagree. J Clin Ethics 1995;639–43.
11. Nitin Ashok John, Jyoti Elgiva John Effective Communication Skills Facilitates Better Health Care Delivery. Br J Pharm Med Res 2022;07(1): 3527–32, January–February 2022. ISSN:2456-9836 Cross Ref DOI: https://doi.org/10.24942/bjpmr.2022.904.
12. Orr RDdeLeon D The role of the clinical ethicist in conflict resolution. J Clin Ethics 2000;1121–30.
13. Quill TE, Brody H. Physician recommendations and patient autonomy: finding a balance between physician power and patient choice. Ann Intern Med 1996;125763–9.
14. Ross N Improving surgical consent. Lancet 2004;364812–3.

**Key Note:** The reader can refer following cases for understanding the true sense of informed consent and also can analyze how legal litigation arises in case of any breach in following the lae.

1. Samira Kohli vs Dr Prabha Manchanda and Anr on 16 January, 2008 (Refer… https://indiankanoon.org/doc/438423/)

2. Krishan Lal Kumar vs Medical Council of India & Ors on 6 February, 2019 (Refer https://indiankanoon.org/doc/40346775/)
3. Baburao Vithal Lohakpure vs Smt. Suniti Devi Singhania ... on 16 August, 2007 (Refer https://indiankanoon.org/doc/116856684/)

**Disclaimer:** All information in chapter **(Module 3.3: The Foundation of Communication especially in relevance to Surgical Informed Consent)** includes but not limited to; and is for information purpose only. The author declares that the sincere attempt has been made to give standard accurate information in the chapter, but it is not a substitute for any legal or professional advice. The reader should seek advice from legal professional if they are seek consultation and advice for any issue associated with communication especially in relevance to surgical informed consent.

## ASSIGNMENT I

Introductory small group session on the principles of communication with focus on administering informed consent.

The students should take note of important point of lecture. Key points are noted in beginning of the lecture

### Focused small group session

Observe the role play and students are divided in groups to observe, criticize and discuss common mistakes in administering informed consent.

**Students can be divided into small groups with Roll Nos 1–10 can participate in Role Play and Roll Nos 11–20 can observe, criticize and discuss common mistakes in administering informed consent. The group leader can discuss:**

**Praveen** Good Morning Doctor, you had called me for admission today for my knee replacement surgery

**Dr Mukund** Ok, go to sister Shanti ... She will get you admitted

**Praveen** Sir, I want to know my treatment plan and my recovery time ...

**Dr Mukund** As a Surgeon I will give you right treatment ... You are laymen … what to know about medicine

**Praveen** Sir Well if Surgery can be avoided ... Any other treatment

**Dr Mukund** Well what you do knowing treatment stuff

**Praveen** You said I have to sign consent form … for what

**Dr Mukund** ... so many patients sign it without asking any thing ... all trust me... why can't you

**Praveen** But ..............................................

**Write observations below:**

## ASSIGNMENT II

**Skills lab sessions:** The students are instructed to perform tasks as detailed below on standardized or regular patients with opportunity for self critique, critique by patient and by facilitator.

**Note:** The students can be divided in group of 8 each [A group leader among 4 students who shall be performing interaction with patient and shall be self critique, another 4 students (A group leader among 4 students)] who shall play role of standardized patient and these students should discuss in group the points to be discussed as critique by patient and eventually the facilitator should discuss the ideal situation.

**Patient's Mother** Doctor Good Morning, I am Neelu, My daughter had a scooter accident.

**Patient (Meera)** Wincing in pain and agony cries ... mummy ... mummy ...

**Orthopedic Surgeon** goes and examines the case in his casualty room.

**Patient's mother** see Mrs Neelu, it looks to be a fracture of foot, we need to do immediate X-ray, followed by ankle fracture fixation surgery ... Well lets see if there is ankle displacement ... doctor murmurs to himself and goes back ... to ... his OPD as rush is heavy.

**Neelu** waiting for the radiology team and nurses to carry Meera for X-ray ...

**Meera** Ma ... Ma ... its paining ... Oh ... I can't bear it ...

**Neelu** after waiting for five minutes gets angry as no one has come yet to attend her daughter.

**Neelu to Orthopedic Surgeon:** Doctor no one yet came for taking Meera for X-ray ... What is next then ... what treatment ... you are planning ... please give some medicine for pain ... too much.

**Orthopedic Surgeon** See ... I am a Doctor ... I will decide ... please don't disturb ... Wait there ... Nurse will take a sign on consent form.

**Neelu** Consent ... what for signature ...

**Orthopedic Surgeon** Nurse will let you ... know ...

**Meera** unbearable ma ...

## Write observation of self-critique

**Critique by patient**

## Critique by patient and by facilitator

**Disclaimer:** All information in chapter **(Module 3.3: The Foundation of Communication)** includes but not limited to; and is for information purpose only. The author declares that the sincere attempt has been made to give standard accurate information in the chapter, but it is not a substitute for any legal or professional advice. The reader should seek advice from legal professional if they are seeking consultation and advice for any issue associated with fiduciary duty.

## ASSESSMENT

**Formative:** Participation in session II and performance in session III may be used as part of formative assessment.

**The teacher should write their assessment report below:**

2. **Summative:** A skill station in which the student may administer informed consent to a standardized patient.

**The students should write their narration here:**

Module

3.4

# Case Studies in Bioethics: Confidentiality

**Background:** This introduces the student to confidentiality and its limits (also see Module 2.5). The case study discussed in the chapter is self-designed for giving insight regarding the topic. The teacher can formulate case study from practical experience or live situation in their setup for teaching concepts to the student.

**Learning Objectives:** The student should be able to:

Identify, discuss and defend medicolegal, sociocultural and ethical issues as it pertains to confidentiality in patient care.

## Key Points

1. The term confidentiality refers to the principle of keeping any information provided by an individual secure and secret from others, as a part of professional obligation and relationship.
2. It is right of every patient to keep information regarding the health, investigative reports, management strategies and prognosis to himself and to the doctor rendering health care exclusively. Doctors need to abide by the right of patient and keep information confidential.
3. Breaches of confidentiality are unwarranted and may lead to loss of trust by patient in the doctor and patient may not feel continuing their treatment with the concerned doctor or may even lead to filling of litigation by patients or their relatives and doctor can be sued for the same.
4. Confidentiality preserves dignity and autonomy right of a person, and it will also prevent misuse of information.
5. All ethical principal as prescribed by NMC Code of Ethics should be followed when information has to be discussed with residents or junior consultant for management of patients.

6. The patient's consent must be taken before for deciding the extent to which information can be disclosed with other consultant when medical advice has to be seeked for further management of the case and importance of sharing vital information in welfare of best medical advice in interest of patient health should be explained to the patient. This also is helpful when a team of consultants are involved in patient care.
7. Privacy along with confidentiality helps an individual to exert his right of autonomy regarding his health.
8. The confidentiality right along with duty obligation permits information sharing in a specified sphere of boundary among the physicians caring for the patient.
9. Due to this provision of confidentially patient is comfortable sharing personal information about his body functions, medical history, etc. with doctors. As information is limited to doctor it does not cause embarrassment.
10. The doctor must not disclose any information regarding to patient's health unless the same is required by law or patient has given consent for the same.
11. As per Norms of National Medical Council Code of Ethics (as specified in Paragraph 2.2 Patience, Delicacy and Secrecy below) the physician/ doctor has to keep information regarding patients' health confidential. It is physician duty to outweigh risk to public then individual and to protect a healthy person against a communicable disease as per law of state regarding intimation in reference to notifiable communicable diseases.
12. The medical practitioner, medical administrators as well as health care catering institution are ethically bound for not disclosing any health information of a patient.

## 2.2 Patience, Delicacy and Secrecy

Patience and delicacy should characterize the physician. Confidences concerning individual or domestic life entrusted by patients to a physician and defects in the disposition or character of patients observed during medical attendance should never be revealed unless their revelation is required by the laws of the state. Sometimes, however, a physician must determine whether his duty to society requires him to employ knowledge, obtained through confidence as a physician, to protect a healthy person against a communicable disease to which he is about to be exposed. In such instance, the physician should act as he would wish another to act toward one of his own family in like circumstances.

(*Reference:* Code of Medical Ethics: https://www.nmc.org.in/rules-regulations/code-of-medical-ethics-regulations-2002)

## BIBLIOGRAPHY

1. Bourke J, Wessely S. Confidentiality. BMJ. 2008 Apr 19;336(7649): 888–91.
2. Mishra NN, Parker LS, Nimgaonkar VL, Deshpande SN. Privacy and the Right to Information Act, 2005. Indian J Med Ethics. 2008 Oct–Dec; 5(4):158–61.
3. O'Brien J, Chantler C. Confidentiality and the duties of care. J Med Ethics 2003;29:36–40.
4. Souhami R, Chalmers S, Collins R, Luker K, Newton J, Silman A, et al. Personal data for the public good: using health information in medical research. London: The Academy of Medical Sciences, 2006.
5. Vigod S, Bell C, Bohnen J. Privacy of patients' information in hospital lifts: observational study. BMJ 2003;327:1024–5.

**Disclaimer:** All information in chapter **(Module 3.4: Case Studies in Bioethics: Confidentiality)** includes but not limited to; and is for information purpose only. The author declares that the sincere attempt has been made to give standard accurate information in the chapter, but it is not a substitute for any legal or professional advice. The reader should seek advice from legal professional if they are seek consultation and advice for any issue associated with confidentiality.

## ASSIGNMENT I: INTRODUCTION OF CASE (1 hour)

Patient Ramesh is 45-year-old male and was diagnosed as a case of tertiary syphilis. He was truck driver by profession and had several incidences of unprotected intercourse with multiple people when on driving duty. Ramesh on investigation was also HIV positive. His wife was pregnant and in third month of pregnancy. Doctor wanted to get his wife tested for HIV. Ramesh fumed over doctor and asked not to do so.

### Points for discussion

1. The primacy of confidentiality in patient care.
2. What does confidentiality entail?
3. When can confidence be breached with whom and how?
4. Confidentiality and diseases that may engender patients and society.

## ASSIGNMENT II: SELF-DIRECTED LEARNING (2 Hours)

The students are instructed to surf through website and note their observations.

## BIBLIOGRAPHY


1. Bourke J, Wessely S. Confidentiality. BMJ. 2008 Apr 19;336(7649): 888–91.
2. Mishra NN, Parker LS, Nimgaonkar VL, Deshpande SN. Privacy and the Right to Information Act, 2005. Indian J Med Ethics. 2008 Oct–Dec; 5(4):158–61.
3. O'Brien J, Chantler C. Confidentiality and the duties of care. J Med Ethics 2003;29:36–40.
4. Souhami R, Chalmers S, Collins R, Luker K, Newton J, Silman A, et al. Personal data for the public good: using health information in medical research. London: The Academy of Medical Sciences, 2006.
5. Vigod S, Bell C, Bohnen J. Privacy of patients' information in hospital lifts: observational study. BMJ 2003;327:1024–5.

## ASSIGNMENT III: ANCHORING LECTURE (1 hour)

The student to attend lecture and write the lecture notes in diary below.

**Key points are highlighted in beginning of the chapter**

## ASSIGNMENT IV: DISCUSSION AND CLOSURE OF CASE (1 hour)

Patient Ramesh is 45-year-old male and was diagnosed as a case of tertiary syphilis. He was truck driver by profession and had several incidences of unprotected intercourse with multiple people when on driving duty. Ramesh on investigation was also HIV positive. His wife was pregnant and in third month of pregnancy. Doctor wanted to get his wife tested for HIV. Ramesh fumed over doctor and asked not to do so.

### Points for discussion

1. **The primacy of confidentiality in patient care.**

   It is right of every patient to keep information regarding the health, investigative reports, management strategies and prognosis to himself and to the doctor rendering health care exclusively. Doctors need to abide by the right of patient and keep information confidential.

   As per Norms of National Medical Council Code of Ethics the physician/doctor has to keep information regarding patients health confidential and can be disclosed when there is a serious and identified risk to a specific person and/or community; or in case of notifiable communicable diseases."

2. **What does confidentiality entail?**

   The term confidentiality refers to the principle of keeping any information provided by an individual secure and secret from others, as a part of professional obligation and relationship.

3. **When can confidence be breached with whom and how?**

   If doctors, medical administrators who maintain medical record or hospital authority disclose patients health and personal information to others it may be considered as breach.

4. **Confidentiality and diseases** that may engender patients and society: These are sexually transmitted diseases such as syphilis, gonorrhea, HIV, etc.

## BIBLIOGRAPHY


1. Bourke J, Wessely S. Confidentiality. BMJ. 2008 Apr 19;336(7649): 888–91.
2. Mishra NN, Parker LS, Nimgaonkar VL, Deshpande SN. Privacy and the Right to Information Act, 2005. Indian J Med Ethics. 2008 Oct–Dec; 5(4):158–61.
3. O'Brien J, Chantler C. Confidentiality and the duties of care. J Med Ethics 2003;29:36–40.

4. Souhami R, Chalmers S, Collins R, Luker K, Newton J, Silman A, et al. Personal data for the public good: using health information in medical research. London: The Academy of Medical Sciences, 2006.
5. Vigod S, Bell C, Bohnen J. Privacy of patients' information in hospital lifts: observational study. BMJ 2003;327:1024–5.

## ASSESSMENT

1. **Formative:** The students may be assessed based on their active participation in the sessions.
2. **Summative:** Short questions on

   1. **What are the instances in which confidentiality of patient information may be breached?**

Module

3.5

# Case Studies in Bioethics: Fiduciary Duty

**Background:** This module on bioethics emphasizes the fiduciary duty. The case study discussed in the chapter is self-designed for giving insight regarding the topic. The teacher can formulate case study from practical experience or live situation in their setup for teaching concepts to the student.

**Learning Objectives:** The student should be able to:

1. Identify, discuss and defend medicolegal, sociocultural, professional and ethical issues as it pertains to the physician–patient relationship (including fiduciary duty).
2. Identify and discuss physician's role and responsibility to society and the community that she/he serves.

## Lecture: Fiduciary Duty

### Key Points

1. Fiduciary duty is duty owed by a fiduciary to the beneficiary and this is of utmost good faith, trust, confidence and candor. This duty obligates a person to act with great honesty and loyalty toward another person and this stands in the best interests of the other person.
2. It also expects a person carrying duty to act in a way which will benefit someone else, especially financially.
3. The person who performs fiduciary duty is called the fiduciary. And this fiduciary duty is owed to a person who is called beneficiary.
4. In a health care setting doctor owes a primary duty which includes fiduciary duties and it comprises duty of care with loyalty, trust, confidentiality, prudence, good faith with duty towards disclosure.

5. The fiduciary principles are applicable in health care as there are potential risk for conflict of interest, and abuse of trust in health care settings.
6. The fiduciary duty responsibility cautious a physician for a limited and restricted behavioral attitude with patients and to extend a constraint relationship in view of financial obligation if something goes wrong while discharging duties.
7. The fiduciary duties in physician–patient relationship are many a time determined in court of law based on general definition of fiduciary and there is lack of a precise analytical framework and guidelines to examine the case in light of health care settings.
8. The physicians may not be able to exert a direct control over patients' property but they can control the medical costs his/ her patients are incurring. The physician may skew and alter the medical advices so that they get financial gains as secondary income by advice supplementary therapy and consultation which may not be necessary. In such cases a physician may be earmarked as fiduciaries with regarding their patients' financial resources.
9. The physicians may be accused at times of receiving kickbacks for breaching of fiduciary obligations to their patients and may have to stand condemned in court of law. The breaches in fiduciary duty conducted by a doctor may impair the patients' property interests by making patient to pay unnecessary costs for his/her treatment and medical care.
10. Many a time when patient is insured; the doctor may keep patient indoor and charge excessively even when patient could have been treated in outpatient department. This is breaching of fiduciary obligations of doctor to their patients as doctor is acting in a way by giving unnecessary treatment for financial gains.
11. The patient may sue a doctor for recovering the cost of medical care from doctor for treatment that was found to be unnecessary, unreasonable and unreimbursable, by a third-party review including the insurer. Under fiduciary principles the law may permit patient to recover medical care costs from the doctor as it stands as a breach of an implied contract not to prescribe unnecessary care.
12. Doctors do have fiduciaries concerns as they are advisors in planning patient management protocol and as a position extend strong influence over patient psyche and at times a doctor may be lured to prescribe certain treatment which may be unnecessary. Though patients have right to decide but due to lack of adequate medical knowledge usually accept what the doctor says.
13. The doctors who pledge to maintain confidentiality and secrecy with respect to patient health and management strategies and this duty of maintaining confidentiality has fiduciary quality, for patients are left with no choice but to have trust in their doctors. This is breaching of fiduciary obligations of doctor if they break the confidentiality of patients secret information on public platform except under state obligation when patients have infectious diseases.

14. Fiduciary relationship between doctor and patient also exist in informed consent cases. If doctor administer treatment which is unnecessary and in addition to what the doctor has discussed with patient there is a breach in informed consent. The breach in informed consent is considered under ambit of medical negligence under court of law. The patient's consent protects the doctor to the extent where doctor has not taken any advantage of the fiduciary position to procure it. Under exceptional circumstances an operating oncosurgeon may have to remove any additional secondary's which was not disclosed to a patient as it might have been missed while interpreting the PET scan; but this act of oncosurgeon was carried in best interest of patient and should not be considered as breach of informed consent. Litigation may occur is such a situation if patient dies after operation but case needs to be appropriately judged under ambit of law.
15. Instructing doctors to strictly adhere to fiduciary principles may stand immensely helpful in delivering effective health care delivery.

## Role of a Physician in Health Care System and Community

The physicians are medically qualified doctors who examine patients, diagnose and treat them. Moreover, they actively participate in health educating their patients and patient's relatives, play active role in implementing national health care programs and ensure preventive measures to prevent spread of any communicable disease or infections especially in time of epidemics.

The physician being multifaceted plays many vital roles while discharging duties as health care provider and these are:

1. **Role as team leader**: The physicians are team leader in hospital setup and play active role in coordinating, directing, communicating, supervising for imparting effective health care delivery.
2. **Treatment and management of disease:** The physician treats and manage the disease in patients as this is their primary duties.
3. **Catering heath delivery:** Physician caters their services at various health centers and these may be primary health centers at village level, secondary health care (at district level hospitals) and tertiary health care (medical colleges and health institute of national importance and higher learning, etc.) settings.
4. **Role in health education:** The physicians also heath educates their team of paramedics, nurses, technicians, multipurpose workers, etc. while managing patients which also help in improving the clinical skills of paramedics.
5. **Role in health economics and as a social entrepreneur:** The physician plans health care delivery in an appropriate,

cost-effective manner in concurrence with the national health care policies. This helps to establish economically viable health care delivery preventing any financial wastage and losses.

6. **Role in generating health care data:** The physician prescribes various investigations for patients and manages patients aiding in their faster recovery. This data generated over the years of investigative findings and management strategies can be analyzed and opined for planning future management strategies.
7. **Role in prevention of diseases:** Physician advice preventive measure strategies to prevent spreading of communicable diseases in the community. Similarly, they promote and recommend lifestyle changes in patients of obesity, diabetes, hypertension, thyroid disease, etc.
8. **Role in improving quality of life and lifespan:** The physician provide therapeutic, curative, preventive and rehabilitative health care services thereby reducing health burden in community and thus eventually improving human quality of life and lifespan of patients.
9. **Role in management of epidemics:** Physician helps in reducing risk of catastrophic situations as in epidemics by timely intervention and management.
10. **Role as a behavioural therapist in community:** The physician practicing with humanistic approach (treating with compassion and care) helps building trust of patients and this has found to be effective in developing confidence, solace and optimistic hope in patient thereby hastening recovery.
11. **Role in building professionalism and respect towards doctor community:** The professionalism in practices by doctors such as abiding by codes of ethics establishes high ethical standards and this helps in looking forwards towards doctors with respect, trust and confidence by community members thus establishing medical profession at high esteem in the community.
12. **Role as trainers of present and future generation of doctors for community:** The physicians provide on job training in teaching as well as service hospitals thus are developing man force for future health care delivery. This also helps in improving the standard of patient care.

13. **Role as authoritative sources on clinical standards:** The physicians continue lifelong learning to update their medical knowledge thus they are looked forward as authoritative sources on clinical standards and practice for diagnosis and management by the community members for seeking consultation if required.
14. **Participation in national health care program:** The physician participates in implementing various national health care programs in community such as family welfare program, national tuberculosis management program, national program for prevention of malaria, leprosy, tuberculosis, etc.
15. **Participating as social workers:** The physician especially provides honorary services in shelter homes, home for the aged, slums, prison, or as a health provider NGO, etc. and thus provides social service to the community.
16. **Role in changing dynamics of the patient health care:** The advancement in scientific technology and innovations (example: telemedicine and employing artificial intelligence) makes it essential for physicians to upgrade to understand and imbibe the changed dynamics of the patient health care and its delivery.
17. **Provides services matching local area health care needs:** The physicians also must match the local area health care needs depending on the disease prevalent in those areas, innovation in machinery methodology of investigative protocols and modified treatment regime of diseases, and state and nations legislative initiatives (applicable laws, Consumer Protection Act).

## BIBLIOGRAPHY


1. Fiduciary Duties: https://www.law.cornell.edu/wex/fiduciary_duty
2. Institute of Medicine (US); Gray BH, (Eds). The New Health Care for Profit: Doctors and Hospitals in a Competitive Environment. Washington (DC): National Academies Press (US); 1983. Secondary Income From Recommended Treatment: Should Fiduciary Principles Constrain Physician Behavior? Available from: https://www.ncbi.nlm.nih.gov/books/NBK216764/
3. Fiduciary Duties: https://assets.hcca-info.org/Portals/0/PDFs/Resources/Conference_Handouts/Regional_Conference/2016/puerto-rico/Muntanerprint2.pdf
4. Hojat M, Gonnella JS, Erdmann JB, Veloski JJ, Xu G. Primary care and non-primary care physicians: a longitudinal study of their similarities. Acad Med 1995; 70:S17–28.

5. Becker S. The tax-exempt board: fiduciary duties in the context of evaluating strategic alternatives and sales transactions. Health Care Law Mon. 2000 Jul:19–26.
6. Peregrine MW, Schwartz JR, Burgdorfer JE, Gordon DC. The fiduciary duties of healthcare directors in the "zone of insolvency". J Health Law. 2002 Spring;35(2):227–62.
7. Emanuel E, Emanuel L. Four models of the physician–patient relationship. JAMA. 1996;267:2221–6.
8. Deber R. Physicians in health care management: 7: the patient–physician partnership: changing roles and the desire for information. Can Med Assoc J 1994;151:171–6.
9. Katz J. The Silent World of Physician and Patient. New York: Free Press; 1984.

**Disclaimer:** All information in chapter **(Module 3.5: Case Studies in Bioethics: Fiduciary Duty)** includes but not limited to; and is for information purpose only. The author declares that the sincere attempt has been made to give standard accurate information in the chapter, but it is not a substitute for any legal or professional advice. The reader should seek advice from legal professional if they are seek consultation and advice for any issue associated with fiduciary duty.

## LEARNING EXPERIENCE

### ASSIGNMENT I: INTRODUCTION OF CASE (1 hour)

The teacher to discuss the case with the students and may give some clues regarding the posed questions.

A gynecologist operated for two hysterectomies, conducted two caesarean deliveries and thereafter conducted 5 vaginal deliveries till 8 pm in night. She attended evening rounds and by 11 pm. She had a Resident Doctor to help her tonight. But as she had fellowship exams next day; the consultant advised the Resident Doctor not to disturb her till morning 5 pm and went up to her residence home upstairs. There was a case of a female patient of obstructed hernia in critical condition and Resident Doctor stood confused but feared to call the Consultant. The patient's relatives got wild and started shouting to call the Senior Doctor … But Resident and Nurses told the relatives to take patient to government hospital as doctor was gynecologist and not a general surgeon. But relatives said name board ... operating surgeon timing ... but treat her ...

## ASSIGNMENT II: SELF-DIRECTED LEARNING (2 hours)

The students may surf through following research paper and write their observations.

1. Hojat M, Gonnella JS, Erdmann JB, Veloski JJ, Xu G. Primary care and non-primary care physicians: a longitudinal study of their similarities. Acad Med 1995;70:S17–28.
2. Becker S. The tax-exempt board: fiduciary duties in the context of evaluating strategic alternatives and sales transactions. Health Care Law Mon. 2000 Jul:19–26.
3. Peregrine MW, Schwartz JR, Burgdorfer JE, Gordon DC. The fiduciary duties of healthcare directors in the "zone of insolvency". J Health Law. 2002 Spring;35(2):227–62.
4. Emanuel E, Emanuel L. Four models of the physician–patient relationship. JAMA. 1996;267:2221–6.

## ASSIGNMENT III: ANCHORING LECTURE (1 hour)

Key notes for lecture are discussed in beginning of the chapter. The student may attend the lecture and take note of important points discussed in lecture.

## ASSIGNMENT IV: DISCUSSION AND CLOSURE OF CASE (1 hour)

**Points for discussion:**

1. **Duty of a doctor.**
   The physicians are medically qualified doctors who examine patients, diagnose and treat them by providing them standard medical care.
2. **The concept of fiduciary duty**
   Fiduciary duty is duty owed by a fiduciary to the beneficiary and this is of utmost good faith, trust, confidence and candor. This duty obligates a person to act with great honesty and loyalty toward another person and this stands in the best interests of the other person.
3. **Balancing personal and professional life**
   It is necessary to draw lines between personal and professional life and as a doctor the gynecologist should attend to duties rather then deciding to rest for her exams. As a qualified medical doctor she could have attended to the patient and provide them the first aid if required and inform them regarding that the case is beyond her specialty and instruct them to go a suitable hospital nearby.
4. **Where to draw the line?**
   Doctor needs to understand the primary duty and fiduciary duty and should not go after any secondary income from prescribing unnecessary treatment, therapies and consultations. There should be no breach in fiduciary obligations of doctor towards the patients.

## ASSESSMENT

1. **Formative:** The student may be assessed based on their active participation in the sessions.
2. **Summative:** Short questions on: What is fiduciary duty?

## READER'S NOTES

# READER'S NOTES

## READER'S NOTES